DEDICATION

This Perfume Review book is dedicated to all the elegant Perfume Reviewers out there who want to keep record of all the different perfumes you want to try.

You are my inspiration for producing books and I'm honored to be a part of keeping all of your Perfume Review notes and records organized.

This journal notebook will help you record your details about the perfumes that you try.

Thoughtfully put together with these sections to record: Fragrance Name, Strength Concentration, Application & Packaging, Initial Impression, Head/ Top Notes, Heart/ Middle Notes, Base Notes, Other Notes, 3rd Party Impressions, Season, Occasion, Day/ Night?, Buy Again? and Ratings.

HOW TO USE THIS BOOK

The purpose of this book is to keep all of your Perfume Review notes all in one place. It will help keep you organized.

This Perfume Review Journal will allow you to accurately document every detail about your perfumes. It's a great way to chart your course as you try new perfumes.

Here are examples of the prompts for you to fill in and write about your experience in this book:

1. Fragrance Name - Write the Name of The Fragrance, The Brand, The Location, The Date & The Cost.
2. Strength Concentration - Check whether it is Parfum, Eau De Parum, Eau De Toilette, Eau De Cologne or Eau Fraiche concentrated.
3. Application & Packaging - How was the packaging and how do you apply the cologne.
4. Initial Impression - Record what your first impression and thoughts were.
5. Head/ Top Notes - Log what you smell at first (introductory).
6. Heart/ Middle Notes - Write what you get a whiff of in the middle when the top evaporates.
7. Base Notes - Record the base smell that lingers on your skin.
8. Other Notes - Log any other important information that you may want to write, such as your favorite part of trying it out, any oils smells, your response, did you like it, list your least favorite part etc.
9. 3rd Party Impressions - What did someone else think of the smell.
10. Season - Is the perfume for a specific season.
11. Occasion - Is the perfume for a specific occasion.
12. Day/ Night? - Do you wear it at night or in the day or does it matter.
13. Buy Again? Would you buy this perfume again.
14. Projection, Longevity & Overall Rating - Give your star rating for each, up to 5 stars.

Enjoy!

Fragrance	
Brand	Location
Date	Cost

☐ Parfum ☐ Eau De Parum ☐ Eau De Toilette
☐ Eau De Cologne ☐ Eau Fraiche

Application?	
Packaging	
Initial Impression	
Head/Top Notes	
Heart/Middle Notes	
Base Notes	
Notes	
3rd Party Impressions	

Season	Day/Night?
Occasion	Buy Again?

Projection ☆☆☆☆☆	Longevity ☆☆☆☆☆

Overall Rating ☆☆☆☆☆

Fragrance	
Brand	Location
Date	Cost

☐ Parfum ☐ Eau De Parum ☐ Eau De Toilette
☐ Eau De Cologne ☐ Eau Fraiche

Application?	
Packaging	
Initial Impression	
Head/Top Notes	
Heart/Middle Notes	
Base Notes	
Notes	
3rd Party Impressions	

Season	Day/Night?
Occasion	Buy Again?

Projection ☆☆☆☆☆	Longevity ☆☆☆☆☆

Overall Rating ☆☆☆☆☆

Fragrance	
Brand	Location
Date	Cost

☐ Parfum ☐ Eau De Parum ☐ Eau De Toilette
☐ Eau De Cologne ☐ Eau Fraiche

Application?
Packaging
Initial Impression
Head/Top Notes
Heart/Middle Notes
Base Notes
Notes
3rd Party Impressions

Season	Day/Night?
Occasion	Buy Again?

Projection ☆☆☆☆☆	Longevity ☆☆☆☆☆

Overall Rating ☆☆☆☆☆

Fragrance	
Brand	Location
Date	Cost

☐ Parfum ☐ Eau De Parum ☐ Eau De Toilette
☐ Eau De Cologne ☐ Eau Fraiche

Application?
Packaging
Initial Impression
Head/Top Notes
Heart/Middle Notes
Base Notes
Notes
3rd Party Impressions

Season	Day/Night?
Occasion	Buy Again?

Projection ☆☆☆☆☆	Longevity ☆☆☆☆☆

Overall Rating ☆☆☆☆☆

Fragrance	
Brand	Location
Date	Cost

☐ Parfum ☐ Eau De Parum ☐ Eau De Toilette
☐ Eau De Cologne ☐ Eau Fraiche

Application?
Packaging
Initial Impression
Head/Top Notes
Heart/Middle Notes
Base Notes
Notes
3rd Party Impressions

Season	Day/Night?
Occasion	Buy Again?

Projection ☆☆☆☆☆	Longevity ☆☆☆☆☆
Overall Rating ☆☆☆☆☆	

Fragrance	
Brand	Location
Date	Cost

☐ Parfum ☐ Eau De Parum ☐ Eau De Toilette
☐ Eau De Cologne ☐ Eau Fraiche

Application?
Packaging
Initial Impression
Head/Top Notes
Heart/Middle Notes
Base Notes
Notes
3rd Party Impressions

Season	Day/Night?
Occasion	Buy Again?

Projection ☆☆☆☆☆	Longevity ☆☆☆☆☆

Overall Rating ☆☆☆☆☆

Fragrance	
Brand	Location
Date	Cost

☐ Parfum ☐ Eau De Parum ☐ Eau De Toilette ☐ Eau De Cologne ☐ Eau Fraiche

Application?	
Packaging	
Initial Impression	
Head/Top Notes	
Heart/Middle Notes	
Base Notes	
Notes	
3rd Party Impressions	

Season	Day/Night?
Occasion	Buy Again?

Projection ☆☆☆☆☆	Longevity ☆☆☆☆☆

Overall Rating ☆☆☆☆☆

Fragrance	
Brand	Location
Date	Cost

□ Parfum □ Eau De Parum □ Eau De Toilette
□ Eau De Cologne □ Eau Fraiche

Application?
Packaging
Initial Impression
Head/Top Notes
Heart/Middle Notes
Base Notes
Notes
3rd Party Impressions

Season	Day/Night?
Occasion	Buy Again?

Projection ☆☆☆☆☆	Longevity ☆☆☆☆☆

Overall Rating ☆☆☆☆☆

Fragrance	
Brand	Location
Date	Cost

☐ Parfum ☐ Eau De Parum ☐ Eau De Toilette
☐ Eau De Cologne ☐ Eau Fraiche

Application?
Packaging
Initial Impression
Head/Top Notes
Heart/Middle Notes
Base Notes
Notes
3rd Party Impressions

Season	Day/Night?
Occasion	Buy Again?

Projection ☆☆☆☆☆	Longevity ☆☆☆☆☆

Overall Rating ☆☆☆☆☆

Fragrance	
Brand	Location
Date	Cost

□ Parfum □ Eau De Parum □ Eau De Toilette
□ Eau De Cologne □ Eau Fraiche

Application?	
Packaging	
Initial Impression	
Head/Top Notes	
Heart/Middle Notes	
Base Notes	
Notes	
3rd Party Impressions	

Season	Day/Night?
Occasion	Buy Again?

Projection ☆☆☆☆☆	Longevity ☆☆☆☆☆

Overall Rating ☆☆☆☆☆

Fragrance	
Brand	Location
Date	Cost

☐ Parfum ☐ Eau De Parum ☐ Eau De Toilette
☐ Eau De Cologne ☐ Eau Fraiche

Application?
Packaging
Initial Impression
Head/Top Notes
Heart/Middle Notes
Base Notes
Notes
3rd Party Impressions

Season	Day/Night?
Occasion	Buy Again?

Projection ☆☆☆☆☆	Longevity ☆☆☆☆☆

Overall Rating ☆☆☆☆☆

Fragrance	
Brand	Location
Date	Cost

□ Parfum □ Eau De Parum □ Eau De Toilette
□ Eau De Cologne □ Eau Fraiche

Application?
Packaging
Initial Impression
Head/Top Notes
Heart/Middle Notes
Base Notes
Notes
3rd Party Impressions

Season	Day/Night?
Occasion	Buy Again?

Projection ☆☆☆☆☆	Longevity ☆☆☆☆☆

Overall Rating ☆☆☆☆☆

Fragrance	
Brand	Location
Date	Cost

☐ Parfum ☐ Eau De Parum ☐ Eau De Toilette
☐ Eau De Cologne ☐ Eau Fraiche

Application?
Packaging
Initial Impression
Head/Top Notes
Heart/Middle Notes
Base Notes
Notes
3rd Party Impressions

Season	Day/Night?
Occasion	Buy Again?

Projection ☆☆☆☆☆	Longevity ☆☆☆☆☆

Overall Rating ☆☆☆☆☆

Fragrance	
Brand	Location
Date	Cost

☐ Parfum ☐ Eau De Parum ☐ Eau De Toilette
☐ Eau De Cologne ☐ Eau Fraiche

Application?
Packaging
Initial Impression
Head/Top Notes
Heart/Middle Notes
Base Notes
Notes
3rd Party Impressions

Season	Day/Night?
Occasion	Buy Again?

Projection ☆☆☆☆☆	Longevity ☆☆☆☆☆

Overall Rating ☆☆☆☆☆

Fragrance	
Brand	Location
Date	Cost

□ Parfum □ Eau De Parum □ Eau De Toilette
□ Eau De Cologne □ Eau Fraiche

Application?
Packaging
Initial Impression
Head/Top Notes
Heart/Middle Notes
Base Notes
Notes
3rd Party Impressions

Season	Day/Night?
Occasion	Buy Again?

Projection ☆☆☆☆☆	Longevity ☆☆☆☆☆

Overall Rating ☆☆☆☆☆

Fragrance	
Brand	Location
Date	Cost

☐ Parfum ☐ Eau De Parum ☐ Eau De Toilette
☐ Eau De Cologne ☐ Eau Fraiche

Application?
Packaging
Initial Impression
Head/Top Notes
Heart/Middle Notes
Base Notes
Notes
3rd Party Impressions

Season	Day/Night?
Occasion	Buy Again?

Projection ☆☆☆☆☆	Longevity ☆☆☆☆☆

Overall Rating ☆☆☆☆☆

Fragrance	
Brand	Location
Date	Cost

☐ Parfum ☐ Eau De Parum ☐ Eau De Toilette
☐ Eau De Cologne ☐ Eau Fraiche

Application?	
Packaging	
Initial Impression	
Head/Top Notes	
Heart/Middle Notes	
Base Notes	
Notes	
3rd Party Impressions	

Season	Day/Night?
Occasion	Buy Again?
Projection ☆☆☆☆☆	Longevity ☆☆☆☆☆

Overall Rating ☆☆☆☆☆

Fragrance	
Brand	Location
Date	Cost

☐ Parfum ☐ Eau De Parum ☐ Eau De Toilette
☐ Eau De Cologne ☐ Eau Fraiche

Application?
Packaging
Initial Impression
Head/Top Notes
Heart/Middle Notes
Base Notes
Notes
3rd Party Impressions

Season	Day/Night?
Occasion	Buy Again?

Projection ☆☆☆☆☆	Longevity ☆☆☆☆☆
Overall Rating ☆☆☆☆☆	

Fragrance	
Brand	Location
Date	Cost

☐ Parfum ☐ Eau De Parum ☐ Eau De Toilette
☐ Eau De Cologne ☐ Eau Fraiche

Application?
Packaging
Initial Impression
Head/Top Notes
Heart/Middle Notes
Base Notes
Notes
3rd Party Impressions

Season	Day/Night?
Occasion	Buy Again?

Projection ☆☆☆☆☆	Longevity ☆☆☆☆☆

Overall Rating ☆☆☆☆☆

Fragrance	
Brand	Location
Date	Cost

□ Parfum □ Eau De Parum □ Eau De Toilette
□ Eau De Cologne □ Eau Fraiche

Application?	
Packaging	
Initial Impression	
Head/Top Notes	
Heart/Middle Notes	
Base Notes	
Notes	
3rd Party Impressions	

Season	Day/Night?
Occasion	Buy Again?

Projection ☆☆☆☆☆	Longevity ☆☆☆☆☆

Overall Rating ☆☆☆☆☆

Fragrance	
Brand	Location
Date	Cost

☐ Parfum ☐ Eau De Parum ☐ Eau De Toilette
☐ Eau De Cologne ☐ Eau Fraiche

Application?
Packaging
Initial Impression
Head/Top Notes
Heart/Middle Notes
Base Notes
Notes
3rd Party Impressions

Season	Day/Night?
Occasion	Buy Again?

Projection ☆☆☆☆☆	Longevity ☆☆☆☆☆

Overall Rating ☆☆☆☆☆

Fragrance	
Brand	Location
Date	Cost

☐ Parfum ☐ Eau De Parum ☐ Eau De Toilette
☐ Eau De Cologne ☐ Eau Fraiche

Application?	
Packaging	
Initial Impression	
Head/Top Notes	
Heart/Middle Notes	
Base Notes	
Notes	
3rd Party Impressions	

Season	Day/Night?
Occasion	Buy Again?

Projection ☆☆☆☆☆	Longevity ☆☆☆☆☆

Overall Rating ☆☆☆☆☆

Fragrance	
Brand	Location
Date	Cost

☐ Parfum ☐ Eau De Parum ☐ Eau De Toilette
☐ Eau De Cologne ☐ Eau Fraiche

Application?	
Packaging	
Initial Impression	
Head/Top Notes	
Heart/Middle Notes	
Base Notes	
Notes	
3rd Party Impressions	

Season	Day/Night?
Occasion	Buy Again?

Projection ☆☆☆☆☆	Longevity ☆☆☆☆☆

Overall Rating ☆☆☆☆☆

Fragrance	
Brand	Location
Date	Cost

☐ Parfum ☐ Eau De Parum ☐ Eau De Toilette
☐ Eau De Cologne ☐ Eau Fraiche

Application?
Packaging
Initial Impression
Head/Top Notes
Heart/Middle Notes
Base Notes
Notes
3rd Party Impressions

Season	Day/Night?
Occasion	Buy Again?

Projection ☆☆☆☆☆	Longevity ☆☆☆☆☆

Overall Rating ☆☆☆☆☆

Fragrance	
Brand	Location
Date	Cost

□ Parfum □ Eau De Parum □ Eau De Toilette
□ Eau De Cologne □ Eau Fraiche

Application?	
Packaging	
Initial Impression	
Head/Top Notes	
Heart/Middle Notes	
Base Notes	
Notes	
3rd Party Impressions	

Season	Day/Night?
Occasion	Buy Again?

Projection ☆☆☆☆☆	Longevity ☆☆☆☆☆

Overall Rating ☆☆☆☆☆

Fragrance	
Brand	Location
Date	Cost

☐ Parfum ☐ Eau De Parum ☐ Eau De Toilette
☐ Eau De Cologne ☐ Eau Fraiche

Application?	
Packaging	
Initial Impression	
Head/Top Notes	
Heart/Middle Notes	
Base Notes	
Notes	
3rd Party Impressions	

Season	Day/Night?
Occasion	Buy Again?

Projection ☆☆☆☆☆	Longevity ☆☆☆☆☆

Overall Rating ☆☆☆☆☆

Fragrance	
Brand	Location
Date	Cost

□ Parfum □ Eau De Parum □ Eau De Toilette
□ Eau De Cologne □ Eau Fraiche

Application?	
Packaging	
Initial Impression	
Head/Top Notes	
Heart/Middle Notes	
Base Notes	
Notes	
3rd Party Impressions	
Season	Day/Night?
Occasion	Buy Again?
Projection ☆☆☆☆☆	Longevity ☆☆☆☆☆

Overall Rating ☆☆☆☆☆

Fragrance	
Brand	Location
Date	Cost

☐ Parfum ☐ Eau De Parum ☐ Eau De Toilette
☐ Eau De Cologne ☐ Eau Fraiche

Application?	
Packaging	
Initial Impression	
Head/Top Notes	
Heart/Middle Notes	
Base Notes	
Notes	
3rd Party Impressions	

Season	Day/Night?
Occasion	Buy Again?

Projection ☆☆☆☆☆	Longevity ☆☆☆☆☆

Overall Rating ☆☆☆☆☆

Fragrance	
Brand	Location
Date	Cost

☐ Parfum ☐ Eau De Parum ☐ Eau De Toilette
☐ Eau De Cologne ☐ Eau Fraiche

Application?	
Packaging	
Initial Impression	
Head/Top Notes	
Heart/Middle Notes	
Base Notes	
Notes	
3rd Party Impressions	

Season	Day/Night?
Occasion	Buy Again?

Projection ☆☆☆☆☆	Longevity ☆☆☆☆☆

Overall Rating ☆☆☆☆☆

Fragrance	
Brand	Location
Date	Cost

☐ Parfum ☐ Eau De Parum ☐ Eau De Toilette
☐ Eau De Cologne ☐ Eau Fraiche

Application?
Packaging
Initial Impression
Head/Top Notes
Heart/Middle Notes
Base Notes
Notes
3rd Party Impressions

Season	Day/Night?
Occasion	Buy Again?

Projection ☆☆☆☆☆	Longevity ☆☆☆☆☆
Overall Rating ☆☆☆☆☆	

Fragrance	
Brand	Location
Date	Cost

☐ Parfum ☐ Eau De Parum ☐ Eau De Toilette
☐ Eau De Cologne ☐ Eau Fraiche

Application?
Packaging
Initial Impression
Head/Top Notes
Heart/Middle Notes
Base Notes
Notes
3rd Party Impressions

Season	Day/Night?
Occasion	Buy Again?
Projection ☆☆☆☆☆	Longevity ☆☆☆☆☆
Overall Rating ☆☆☆☆☆	

Fragrance	
Brand	Location
Date	Cost

☐ Parfum ☐ Eau De Parum ☐ Eau De Toilette
☐ Eau De Cologne ☐ Eau Fraiche

Application?
Packaging
Initial Impression
Head/Top Notes
Heart/Middle Notes
Base Notes
Notes
3rd Party Impressions

Season	Day/Night?
Occasion	Buy Again?

Projection ☆☆☆☆☆	Longevity ☆☆☆☆☆

Overall Rating ☆☆☆☆☆

Fragrance	
Brand	Location
Date	Cost

☐ Parfum ☐ Eau De Parum ☐ Eau De Toilette
☐ Eau De Cologne ☐ Eau Fraiche

Application?
Packaging
Initial Impression
Head/Top Notes
Heart/Middle Notes
Base Notes
Notes
3rd Party Impressions

Season	Day/Night?
Occasion	Buy Again?

Projection ☆☆☆☆☆	Longevity ☆☆☆☆☆
Overall Rating ☆☆☆☆☆	

Fragrance	
Brand	Location
Date	Cost

☐ Parfum ☐ Eau De Parum ☐ Eau De Toilette
☐ Eau De Cologne ☐ Eau Fraiche

Application?
Packaging
Initial Impression
Head/Top Notes
Heart/Middle Notes
Base Notes
Notes
3rd Party Impressions

Season	Day/Night?
Occasion	Buy Again?

Projection ☆☆☆☆☆	Longevity ☆☆☆☆☆

Overall Rating ☆☆☆☆☆

Fragrance	
Brand	Location
Date	Cost

□ Parfum □ Eau De Parum □ Eau De Toilette
□ Eau De Cologne □ Eau Fraiche

Application?
Packaging
Initial Impression
Head/Top Notes
Heart/Middle Notes
Base Notes
Notes
3rd Party Impressions

Season	Day/Night?
Occasion	Buy Again?
Projection ☆☆☆☆☆	Longevity ☆☆☆☆☆

Overall Rating ☆☆☆☆☆

Fragrance	
Brand	Location
Date	Cost

☐ Parfum ☐ Eau De Parum ☐ Eau De Toilette
☐ Eau De Cologne ☐ Eau Fraiche

Application?
Packaging
Initial Impression
Head/Top Notes
Heart/Middle Notes
Base Notes
Notes
3rd Party Impressions

Season	Day/Night?
Occasion	Buy Again?

Projection ☆☆☆☆☆	Longevity ☆☆☆☆☆

Overall Rating ☆☆☆☆☆

Fragrance	
Brand	Location
Date	Cost

☐ Parfum ☐ Eau De Parum ☐ Eau De Toilette
☐ Eau De Cologne ☐ Eau Fraiche

Application?
Packaging
Initial Impression
Head/Top Notes
Heart/Middle Notes
Base Notes
Notes
3rd Party Impressions

Season	Day/Night?
Occasion	Buy Again?

Projection ☆☆☆☆☆	Longevity ☆☆☆☆☆

Overall Rating ☆☆☆☆☆

Fragrance	
Brand	Location
Date	Cost

☐ Parfum ☐ Eau De Parum ☐ Eau De Toilette
☐ Eau De Cologne ☐ Eau Fraiche

Application?
Packaging
Initial Impression
Head/Top Notes
Heart/Middle Notes
Base Notes
Notes
3rd Party Impressions

Season	Day/Night?
Occasion	Buy Again?

Projection ☆☆☆☆☆	Longevity ☆☆☆☆☆

Overall Rating ☆☆☆☆☆

Fragrance	
Brand	Location
Date	Cost

☐ Parfum ☐ Eau De Parum ☐ Eau De Toilette
☐ Eau De Cologne ☐ Eau Fraiche

Application?
Packaging
Initial Impression
Head/Top Notes
Heart/Middle Notes
Base Notes
Notes
3rd Party Impressions

Season	Day/Night?
Occasion	Buy Again?

Projection ☆☆☆☆☆	Longevity ☆☆☆☆☆

Overall Rating ☆☆☆☆☆

Fragrance	
Brand	Location
Date	Cost

□ Parfum □ Eau De Parum □ Eau De Toilette
□ Eau De Cologne □ Eau Fraiche

Application?
Packaging
Initial Impression
Head/Top Notes
Heart/Middle Notes
Base Notes
Notes
3rd Party Impressions

Season	Day/Night?
Occasion	Buy Again?

Projection ☆☆☆☆☆	Longevity ☆☆☆☆☆

Overall Rating ☆☆☆☆☆

Fragrance	
Brand	Location
Date	Cost

☐ Parfum ☐ Eau De Parum ☐ Eau De Toilette
☐ Eau De Cologne ☐ Eau Fraiche

Application?	
Packaging	
Initial Impression	
Head/Top Notes	
Heart/Middle Notes	
Base Notes	
Notes	
3rd Party Impressions	

Season	Day/Night?
Occasion	Buy Again?

Projection ☆☆☆☆☆	Longevity ☆☆☆☆☆

Overall Rating ☆☆☆☆☆

Fragrance	
Brand	Location
Date	Cost

☐ Parfum ☐ Eau De Parum ☐ Eau De Toilette
☐ Eau De Cologne ☐ Eau Fraiche

Application?
Packaging
Initial Impression
Head/Top Notes
Heart/Middle Notes
Base Notes
Notes
3rd Party Impressions

Season	Day/Night?
Occasion	Buy Again?

Projection ☆☆☆☆☆	Longevity ☆☆☆☆☆

Overall Rating ☆☆☆☆☆

Fragrance	
Brand	Location
Date	Cost

☐ Parfum ☐ Eau De Parum ☐ Eau De Toilette
☐ Eau De Cologne ☐ Eau Fraiche

Application?
Packaging
Initial Impression
Head/Top Notes
Heart/Middle Notes
Base Notes
Notes
3rd Party Impressions

Season	Day/Night?
Occasion	Buy Again?
Projection ☆☆☆☆☆	Longevity ☆☆☆☆☆

Overall Rating ☆☆☆☆☆

Fragrance	
Brand	Location
Date	Cost

☐ Parfum ☐ Eau De Parum ☐ Eau De Toilette
☐ Eau De Cologne ☐ Eau Fraiche

Application?
Packaging
Initial Impression
Head/Top Notes
Heart/Middle Notes
Base Notes
Notes
3rd Party Impressions

Season	Day/Night?
Occasion	Buy Again?

Projection ☆☆☆☆☆	Longevity ☆☆☆☆☆

Overall Rating ☆☆☆☆☆

Fragrance	
Brand	Location
Date	Cost

□ Parfum □ Eau De Parum □ Eau De Toilette
□ Eau De Cologne □ Eau Fraiche

Application?
Packaging
Initial Impression
Head/Top Notes
Heart/Middle Notes
Base Notes
Notes
3rd Party Impressions

Season	Day/Night?
Occasion	Buy Again?

Projection ☆☆☆☆☆	Longevity ☆☆☆☆☆

Overall Rating ☆☆☆☆☆

Fragrance	
Brand	Location
Date	Cost

☐ Parfum ☐ Eau De Parum ☐ Eau De Toilette
☐ Eau De Cologne ☐ Eau Fraiche

Application?
Packaging
Initial Impression
Head/Top Notes
Heart/Middle Notes
Base Notes
Notes
3rd Party Impressions

Season	Day/Night?
Occasion	Buy Again?

Projection ☆☆☆☆☆	Longevity ☆☆☆☆☆

Overall Rating ☆☆☆☆☆

Fragrance	
Brand	Location
Date	Cost

☐ Parfum ☐ Eau De Parum ☐ Eau De Toilette
☐ Eau De Cologne ☐ Eau Fraiche

Application?
Packaging
Initial Impression
Head/Top Notes
Heart/Middle Notes
Base Notes
Notes
3rd Party Impressions

Season	Day/Night?
Occasion	Buy Again?

Projection ☆☆☆☆☆	Longevity ☆☆☆☆☆

Overall Rating ☆☆☆☆☆

Fragrance	
Brand	Location
Date	Cost

☐ Parfum ☐ Eau De Parum ☐ Eau De Toilette ☐ Eau De Cologne ☐ Eau Fraiche

Application?
Packaging
Initial Impression
Head/Top Notes
Heart/Middle Notes
Base Notes
Notes
3rd Party Impressions

Season	Day/Night?
Occasion	Buy Again?

Projection ☆☆☆☆☆	Longevity ☆☆☆☆☆

Overall Rating ☆☆☆☆☆

Fragrance	
Brand	Location
Date	Cost

☐ Parfum ☐ Eau De Parum ☐ Eau De Toilette
☐ Eau De Cologne ☐ Eau Fraiche

Application?
Packaging
Initial Impression
Head/Top Notes
Heart/Middle Notes
Base Notes
Notes
3rd Party Impressions

Season	Day/Night?
Occasion	Buy Again?

Projection ☆☆☆☆☆	Longevity ☆☆☆☆☆

Overall Rating ☆☆☆☆☆

Fragrance	
Brand	Location
Date	Cost

☐ Parfum ☐ Eau De Parum ☐ Eau De Toilette
☐ Eau De Cologne ☐ Eau Fraiche

Application?	
Packaging	
Initial Impression	
Head/Top Notes	
Heart/Middle Notes	
Base Notes	
Notes	
3rd Party Impressions	

Season	Day/Night?
Occasion	Buy Again?

Projection ☆☆☆☆☆	Longevity ☆☆☆☆☆

Overall Rating ☆☆☆☆☆

Fragrance	
Brand	Location
Date	Cost

☐ Parfum ☐ Eau De Parum ☐ Eau De Toilette
☐ Eau De Cologne ☐ Eau Fraiche

Application?
Packaging
Initial Impression
Head/Top Notes
Heart/Middle Notes
Base Notes
Notes
3rd Party Impressions

Season	Day/Night?
Occasion	Buy Again?

Projection ☆☆☆☆☆	Longevity ☆☆☆☆☆

Overall Rating ☆☆☆☆☆

Fragrance	
Brand	Location
Date	Cost

☐ Parfum ☐ Eau De Parum ☐ Eau De Toilette
☐ Eau De Cologne ☐ Eau Fraiche

Application?
Packaging
Initial Impression
Head/Top Notes
Heart/Middle Notes
Base Notes
Notes
3rd Party Impressions

Season	Day/Night?
Occasion	Buy Again?

Projection ☆☆☆☆☆	Longevity ☆☆☆☆☆

Overall Rating ☆☆☆☆☆

Fragrance	
Brand	Location
Date	Cost

☐ Parfum ☐ Eau De Parum ☐ Eau De Toilette
☐ Eau De Cologne ☐ Eau Fraiche

Application?	
Packaging	
Initial Impression	
Head/Top Notes	
Heart/Middle Notes	
Base Notes	
Notes	
3rd Party Impressions	

Season	Day/Night?
Occasion	Buy Again?

Projection ☆☆☆☆☆	Longevity ☆☆☆☆☆

Overall Rating ☆☆☆☆☆

Fragrance	
Brand	Location
Date	Cost

☐ Parfum ☐ Eau De Parum ☐ Eau De Toilette
☐ Eau De Cologne ☐ Eau Fraiche

Application?
Packaging
Initial Impression
Head/Top Notes
Heart/Middle Notes
Base Notes
Notes
3rd Party Impressions

Season	Day/Night?
Occasion	Buy Again?

Projection ☆☆☆☆☆	Longevity ☆☆☆☆☆

Overall Rating ☆☆☆☆☆

Fragrance	
Brand	Location
Date	Cost

☐ Parfum ☐ Eau De Parum ☐ Eau De Toilette
☐ Eau De Cologne ☐ Eau Fraiche

Application?
Packaging
Initial Impression
Head/Top Notes
Heart/Middle Notes
Base Notes
Notes
3rd Party Impressions

Season	Day/Night?
Occasion	Buy Again?

Projection ☆☆☆☆☆	Longevity ☆☆☆☆☆

Overall Rating ☆☆☆☆☆

Fragrance	
Brand	Location
Date	Cost

☐ Parfum ☐ Eau De Parum ☐ Eau De Toilette
☐ Eau De Cologne ☐ Eau Fraiche

Application?
Packaging
Initial Impression
Head/Top Notes
Heart/Middle Notes
Base Notes
Notes
3rd Party Impressions

Season	Day/Night?
Occasion	Buy Again?

Projection ☆☆☆☆☆	Longevity ☆☆☆☆☆

Overall Rating ☆☆☆☆☆

Fragrance	
Brand	Location
Date	Cost

☐ Parfum ☐ Eau De Parum ☐ Eau De Toilette
☐ Eau De Cologne ☐ Eau Fraiche

Application?
Packaging
Initial Impression
Head/Top Notes
Heart/Middle Notes
Base Notes
Notes
3rd Party Impressions

Season	Day/Night?
Occasion	Buy Again?
Projection ☆☆☆☆☆	Longevity ☆☆☆☆☆

Overall Rating ☆☆☆☆☆

Fragrance	
Brand	Location
Date	Cost

☐ Parfum ☐ Eau De Parum ☐ Eau De Toilette
☐ Eau De Cologne ☐ Eau Fraiche

Application?
Packaging
Initial Impression
Head/Top Notes
Heart/Middle Notes
Base Notes
Notes
3rd Party Impressions

Season	Day/Night?
Occasion	Buy Again?

Projection ☆☆☆☆☆	Longevity ☆☆☆☆☆

Overall Rating ☆☆☆☆☆

Fragrance	
Brand	Location
Date	Cost

□ Parfum □ Eau De Parum □ Eau De Toilette
□ Eau De Cologne □ Eau Fraiche

Application?
Packaging
Initial Impression
Head/Top Notes
Heart/Middle Notes
Base Notes
Notes
3rd Party Impressions

Season	Day/Night?
Occasion	Buy Again?
Projection ☆☆☆☆☆	Longevity ☆☆☆☆☆

Overall Rating ☆☆☆☆☆

Fragrance	
Brand	Location
Date	Cost

□ Parfum □ Eau De Parum □ Eau De Toilette
□ Eau De Cologne □ Eau Fraiche

Application?	
Packaging	
Initial Impression	
Head/Top Notes	
Heart/Middle Notes	
Base Notes	
Notes	
3rd Party Impressions	

Season	Day/Night?
Occasion	Buy Again?

Projection ☆☆☆☆☆	Longevity ☆☆☆☆☆

Overall Rating ☆☆☆☆☆

Fragrance	
Brand	Location
Date	Cost

☐ Parfum ☐ Eau De Parum ☐ Eau De Toilette
☐ Eau De Cologne ☐ Eau Fraiche

Application?	
Packaging	
Initial Impression	
Head/Top Notes	
Heart/Middle Notes	
Base Notes	
Notes	
3rd Party Impressions	

Season	Day/Night?
Occasion	Buy Again?

Projection ☆☆☆☆☆	Longevity ☆☆☆☆☆

Overall Rating ☆☆☆☆☆

Fragrance	
Brand	Location
Date	Cost

□ Parfum □ Eau De Parum □ Eau De Toilette
□ Eau De Cologne □ Eau Fraiche

Application?	
Packaging	
Initial Impression	
Head/Top Notes	
Heart/Middle Notes	
Base Notes	
Notes	
3rd Party Impressions	

Season	Day/Night?
Occasion	Buy Again?

Projection ☆☆☆☆☆	Longevity ☆☆☆☆☆

Overall Rating ☆☆☆☆☆

Fragrance	
Brand	Location
Date	Cost

☐ Parfum ☐ Eau De Parum ☐ Eau De Toilette
☐ Eau De Cologne ☐ Eau Fraiche

Application?
Packaging
Initial Impression
Head/Top Notes
Heart/Middle Notes
Base Notes
Notes
3rd Party Impressions

Season	Day/Night?
Occasion	Buy Again?
Projection ☆☆☆☆☆	Longevity ☆☆☆☆☆

Overall Rating ☆☆☆☆☆

Fragrance	
Brand	Location
Date	Cost

☐ Parfum ☐ Eau De Parum ☐ Eau De Toilette
☐ Eau De Cologne ☐ Eau Fraiche

Application?	
Packaging	
Initial Impression	
Head/Top Notes	
Heart/Middle Notes	
Base Notes	
Notes	
3rd Party Impressions	

Season	Day/Night?
Occasion	Buy Again?

Projection ☆☆☆☆☆	Longevity ☆☆☆☆☆

Overall Rating ☆☆☆☆☆

Fragrance	
Brand	Location
Date	Cost

□ Parfum □ Eau De Parum □ Eau De Toilette □ Eau De Cologne □ Eau Fraiche

Application?	
Packaging	
Initial Impression	
Head/Top Notes	
Heart/Middle Notes	
Base Notes	
Notes	
3rd Party Impressions	

Season	Day/Night?
Occasion	Buy Again?

Projection ☆☆☆☆☆	Longevity ☆☆☆☆☆

Overall Rating ☆☆☆☆☆

Fragrance	
Brand	Location
Date	Cost

☐ Parfum ☐ Eau De Parum ☐ Eau De Toilette
☐ Eau De Cologne ☐ Eau Fraiche

Application?
Packaging
Initial Impression
Head/Top Notes
Heart/Middle Notes
Base Notes
Notes
3rd Party Impressions

Season	Day/Night?
Occasion	Buy Again?

Projection ☆☆☆☆☆	Longevity ☆☆☆☆☆

Overall Rating ☆☆☆☆☆

Fragrance	
Brand	Location
Date	Cost

☐ Parfum ☐ Eau De Parum ☐ Eau De Toilette
☐ Eau De Cologne ☐ Eau Fraiche

Application?	
Packaging	
Initial Impression	
Head/Top Notes	
Heart/Middle Notes	
Base Notes	
Notes	
3rd Party Impressions	

Season	Day/Night?
Occasion	Buy Again?

Projection ☆☆☆☆☆	Longevity ☆☆☆☆☆

Overall Rating ☆☆☆☆☆

Fragrance	
Brand	Location
Date	Cost

☐ Parfum ☐ Eau De Parum ☐ Eau De Toilette
☐ Eau De Cologne ☐ Eau Fraiche

Application?
Packaging
Initial Impression
Head/Top Notes
Heart/Middle Notes
Base Notes
Notes
3rd Party Impressions

Season	Day/Night?
Occasion	Buy Again?

Projection ☆☆☆☆☆	Longevity ☆☆☆☆☆

Overall Rating ☆☆☆☆☆

Fragrance	
Brand	Location
Date	Cost

☐ Parfum ☐ Eau De Parum ☐ Eau De Toilette
☐ Eau De Cologne ☐ Eau Fraiche

Application?
Packaging
Initial Impression
Head/Top Notes
Heart/Middle Notes
Base Notes
Notes
3rd Party Impressions

Season	Day/Night?
Occasion	Buy Again?

Projection ☆☆☆☆☆	Longevity ☆☆☆☆☆

Overall Rating ☆☆☆☆☆

Fragrance	
Brand	Location
Date	Cost

☐ Parfum ☐ Eau De Parum ☐ Eau De Toilette
☐ Eau De Cologne ☐ Eau Fraiche

Application?
Packaging
Initial Impression
Head/Top Notes
Heart/Middle Notes
Base Notes
Notes
3rd Party Impressions

Season	Day/Night?
Occasion	Buy Again?

Projection ☆☆☆☆☆	Longevity ☆☆☆☆☆

Overall Rating ☆☆☆☆☆

Fragrance	
Brand	Location
Date	Cost

☐ Parfum ☐ Eau De Parum ☐ Eau De Toilette
☐ Eau De Cologne ☐ Eau Fraiche

Application?	
Packaging	
Initial Impression	
Head/Top Notes	
Heart/Middle Notes	
Base Notes	
Notes	
3rd Party Impressions	

Season	Day/Night?
Occasion	Buy Again?

Projection ☆☆☆☆☆	Longevity ☆☆☆☆☆

Overall Rating ☆☆☆☆☆

Fragrance	
Brand	Location
Date	Cost

☐ Parfum ☐ Eau De Parum ☐ Eau De Toilette
☐ Eau De Cologne ☐ Eau Fraiche

Application?	
Packaging	
Initial Impression	
Head/Top Notes	
Heart/Middle Notes	
Base Notes	
Notes	
3rd Party Impressions	

Season	Day/Night?
Occasion	Buy Again?

Projection ☆☆☆☆☆	Longevity ☆☆☆☆☆

Overall Rating ☆☆☆☆☆

Fragrance	
Brand	Location
Date	Cost

☐ Parfum ☐ Eau De Parum ☐ Eau De Toilette
☐ Eau De Cologne ☐ Eau Fraiche

Application?	
Packaging	
Initial Impression	
Head/Top Notes	
Heart/Middle Notes	
Base Notes	
Notes	
3rd Party Impressions	

Season	Day/Night?
Occasion	Buy Again?

Projection ☆☆☆☆☆	Longevity ☆☆☆☆☆

Overall Rating ☆☆☆☆☆

Fragrance	
Brand	Location
Date	Cost

☐ Parfum ☐ Eau De Parum ☐ Eau De Toilette
☐ Eau De Cologne ☐ Eau Fraiche

Application?	
Packaging	
Initial Impression	
Head/Top Notes	
Heart/Middle Notes	
Base Notes	
Notes	
3rd Party Impressions	

Season	Day/Night?
Occasion	Buy Again?

Projection ☆☆☆☆☆	Longevity ☆☆☆☆☆

Overall Rating ☆☆☆☆☆

Fragrance	
Brand	Location
Date	Cost

☐ Parfum ☐ Eau De Parum ☐ Eau De Toilette
☐ Eau De Cologne ☐ Eau Fraiche

Application?	
Packaging	
Initial Impression	
Head/Top Notes	
Heart/Middle Notes	
Base Notes	
Notes	
3rd Party Impressions	

Season	Day/Night?
Occasion	Buy Again?

Projection ☆☆☆☆☆	Longevity ☆☆☆☆☆

Overall Rating ☆☆☆☆☆

Fragrance	
Brand	Location
Date	Cost

□ Parfum □ Eau De Parum □ Eau De Toilette
□ Eau De Cologne □ Eau Fraiche

Application?
Packaging
Initial Impression
Head/Top Notes
Heart/Middle Notes
Base Notes
Notes
3rd Party Impressions

Season	Day/Night?
Occasion	Buy Again?

Projection ☆☆☆☆☆	Longevity ☆☆☆☆☆

Overall Rating ☆☆☆☆☆

Fragrance	
Brand	Location
Date	Cost

☐ Parfum ☐ Eau De Parum ☐ Eau De Toilette
☐ Eau De Cologne ☐ Eau Fraiche

Application?	
Packaging	
Initial Impression	
Head/Top Notes	
Heart/Middle Notes	
Base Notes	
Notes	
3rd Party Impressions	

Season	Day/Night?
Occasion	Buy Again?

Projection ☆☆☆☆☆	Longevity ☆☆☆☆☆

Overall Rating ☆☆☆☆☆

Fragrance	
Brand	Location
Date	Cost

☐ Parfum ☐ Eau De Parum ☐ Eau De Toilette
☐ Eau De Cologne ☐ Eau Fraiche

Application?	
Packaging	
Initial Impression	
Head/Top Notes	
Heart/Middle Notes	
Base Notes	
Notes	
3rd Party Impressions	

Season	Day/Night?
Occasion	Buy Again?

Projection ☆☆☆☆☆	Longevity ☆☆☆☆☆

Overall Rating ☆☆☆☆☆

Fragrance	
Brand	Location
Date	Cost

☐ Parfum ☐ Eau De Parum ☐ Eau De Toilette
☐ Eau De Cologne ☐ Eau Fraiche

Application?
Packaging
Initial Impression
Head/Top Notes
Heart/Middle Notes
Base Notes
Notes
3rd Party Impressions

Season	Day/Night?
Occasion	Buy Again?

Projection ☆☆☆☆☆	Longevity ☆☆☆☆☆

Overall Rating ☆☆☆☆☆

Fragrance	
Brand	Location
Date	Cost

□ Parfum □ Eau De Parum □ Eau De Toilette
□ Eau De Cologne □ Eau Fraiche

Application?
Packaging
Initial Impression
Head/Top Notes
Heart/Middle Notes
Base Notes
Notes
3rd Party Impressions

Season	Day/Night?
Occasion	Buy Again?

Projection ☆☆☆☆☆	Longevity ☆☆☆☆☆

Overall Rating ☆☆☆☆☆

Fragrance	
Brand	Location
Date	Cost

☐ Parfum ☐ Eau De Parum ☐ Eau De Toilette
☐ Eau De Cologne ☐ Eau Fraiche

Application?
Packaging
Initial Impression
Head/Top Notes
Heart/Middle Notes
Base Notes
Notes
3rd Party Impressions

Season	Day/Night?
Occasion	Buy Again?
Projection ☆☆☆☆☆	Longevity ☆☆☆☆☆
Overall Rating ☆☆☆☆☆	

Fragrance	
Brand	Location
Date	Cost

☐ Parfum ☐ Eau De Parum ☐ Eau De Toilette
☐ Eau De Cologne ☐ Eau Fraiche

Application?	
Packaging	
Initial Impression	
Head/Top Notes	
Heart/Middle Notes	
Base Notes	
Notes	
3rd Party Impressions	
Season	Day/Night?
Occasion	Buy Again?

Projection ☆☆☆☆☆	Longevity ☆☆☆☆☆

Overall Rating ☆☆☆☆☆

Fragrance	
Brand	Location
Date	Cost

☐ Parfum ☐ Eau De Parum ☐ Eau De Toilette
☐ Eau De Cologne ☐ Eau Fraiche

Application?
Packaging
Initial Impression
Head/Top Notes
Heart/Middle Notes
Base Notes
Notes
3rd Party Impressions

Season	Day/Night?
Occasion	Buy Again?

Projection ☆☆☆☆☆	Longevity ☆☆☆☆☆

Overall Rating ☆☆☆☆☆

Fragrance	
Brand	Location
Date	Cost

☐ Parfum ☐ Eau De Parum ☐ Eau De Toilette
☐ Eau De Cologne ☐ Eau Fraiche

Application?
Packaging
Initial Impression
Head/Top Notes
Heart/Middle Notes
Base Notes
Notes
3rd Party Impressions

Season	Day/Night?
Occasion	Buy Again?

Projection ☆☆☆☆☆	Longevity ☆☆☆☆☆

Overall Rating ☆☆☆☆☆

Fragrance	
Brand	Location
Date	Cost

☐ Parfum ☐ Eau De Parum ☐ Eau De Toilette
☐ Eau De Cologne ☐ Eau Fraiche

Application?
Packaging
Initial Impression
Head/Top Notes
Heart/Middle Notes
Base Notes
Notes
3rd Party Impressions

Season	Day/Night?
Occasion	Buy Again?

Projection ☆☆☆☆☆	Longevity ☆☆☆☆☆

Overall Rating ☆☆☆☆☆

Fragrance	
Brand	Location
Date	Cost

☐ Parfum ☐ Eau De Parum ☐ Eau De Toilette
☐ Eau De Cologne ☐ Eau Fraiche

Application?
Packaging
Initial Impression
Head/Top Notes
Heart/Middle Notes
Base Notes
Notes
3rd Party Impressions

Season	Day/Night?
Occasion	Buy Again?

Projection ☆☆☆☆☆	Longevity ☆☆☆☆☆

Overall Rating ☆☆☆☆☆

Fragrance	
Brand	Location
Date	Cost

☐ Parfum ☐ Eau De Parum ☐ Eau De Toilette
☐ Eau De Cologne ☐ Eau Fraiche

Application?
Packaging
Initial Impression
Head/Top Notes
Heart/Middle Notes
Base Notes
Notes
3rd Party Impressions

Season	Day/Night?
Occasion	Buy Again?

Projection ☆☆☆☆☆	Longevity ☆☆☆☆☆

Overall Rating ☆☆☆☆☆

Fragrance	
Brand	Location
Date	Cost

☐ Parfum ☐ Eau De Parum ☐ Eau De Toilette
☐ Eau De Cologne ☐ Eau Fraiche

Application?
Packaging
Initial Impression
Head/Top Notes
Heart/Middle Notes
Base Notes
Notes
3rd Party Impressions

Season	Day/Night?
Occasion	Buy Again?

Projection ☆☆☆☆☆	Longevity ☆☆☆☆☆

Overall Rating ☆☆☆☆☆

Fragrance	
Brand	Location
Date	Cost

☐ Parfum ☐ Eau De Parum ☐ Eau De Toilette
☐ Eau De Cologne ☐ Eau Fraiche

Application?
Packaging
Initial Impression
Head/Top Notes
Heart/Middle Notes
Base Notes
Notes
3rd Party Impressions

Season	Day/Night?
Occasion	Buy Again?

Projection ☆☆☆☆☆	Longevity ☆☆☆☆☆

Overall Rating ☆☆☆☆☆

Fragrance	
Brand	Location
Date	Cost

☐ Parfum ☐ Eau De Parum ☐ Eau De Toilette
☐ Eau De Cologne ☐ Eau Fraiche

Application?
Packaging
Initial Impression
Head/Top Notes
Heart/Middle Notes
Base Notes
Notes
3rd Party Impressions

Season	Day/Night?
Occasion	Buy Again?

Projection ☆☆☆☆☆	Longevity ☆☆☆☆☆

Overall Rating ☆☆☆☆☆

Fragrance	
Brand	Location
Date	Cost

☐ Parfum ☐ Eau De Parum ☐ Eau De Toilette
☐ Eau De Cologne ☐ Eau Fraiche

Application?
Packaging
Initial Impression
Head/Top Notes
Heart/Middle Notes
Base Notes
Notes
3rd Party Impressions

Season	Day/Night?
Occasion	Buy Again?

Projection ☆☆☆☆☆	Longevity ☆☆☆☆☆

Overall Rating ☆☆☆☆☆

Fragrance	
Brand	Location
Date	Cost

☐ Parfum ☐ Eau De Parum ☐ Eau De Toilette
☐ Eau De Cologne ☐ Eau Fraiche

Application?
Packaging
Initial Impression
Head/Top Notes
Heart/Middle Notes
Base Notes
Notes
3rd Party Impressions

Season	Day/Night?
Occasion	Buy Again?

Projection ☆☆☆☆☆	Longevity ☆☆☆☆☆

Overall Rating ☆☆☆☆☆

Fragrance	
Brand	Location
Date	Cost

☐ Parfum ☐ Eau De Parum ☐ Eau De Toilette
☐ Eau De Cologne ☐ Eau Fraiche

Application?
Packaging
Initial Impression
Head/Top Notes
Heart/Middle Notes
Base Notes
Notes
3rd Party Impressions

Season	Day/Night?
Occasion	Buy Again?

Projection ☆☆☆☆☆	Longevity ☆☆☆☆☆

Overall Rating ☆☆☆☆☆

Fragrance	
Brand	Location
Date	Cost

☐ Parfum ☐ Eau De Parum ☐ Eau De Toilette
☐ Eau De Cologne ☐ Eau Fraiche

Application?
Packaging
Initial Impression
Head/Top Notes
Heart/Middle Notes
Base Notes
Notes
3rd Party Impressions

Season	Day/Night?
Occasion	Buy Again?

Projection ☆☆☆☆☆	Longevity ☆☆☆☆☆

Overall Rating ☆☆☆☆☆

Fragrance	
Brand	Location
Date	Cost

☐ Parfum ☐ Eau De Parum ☐ Eau De Toilette
☐ Eau De Cologne ☐ Eau Fraiche

Application?	
Packaging	
Initial Impression	
Head/Top Notes	
Heart/Middle Notes	
Base Notes	
Notes	
3rd Party Impressions	

Season	Day/Night?
Occasion	Buy Again?

Projection ☆☆☆☆☆	Longevity ☆☆☆☆☆

Overall Rating ☆☆☆☆☆

Fragrance	
Brand	Location
Date	Cost

☐ Parfum ☐ Eau De Parum ☐ Eau De Toilette
☐ Eau De Cologne ☐ Eau Fraiche

Application?
Packaging
Initial Impression
Head/Top Notes
Heart/Middle Notes
Base Notes
Notes
3rd Party Impressions

Season	Day/Night?
Occasion	Buy Again?

Projection ☆☆☆☆☆	Longevity ☆☆☆☆☆

Overall Rating ☆☆☆☆☆

Fragrance	
Brand	Location
Date	Cost

☐ Parfum ☐ Eau De Parum ☐ Eau De Toilette
☐ Eau De Cologne ☐ Eau Fraiche

Application?
Packaging
Initial Impression
Head/Top Notes
Heart/Middle Notes
Base Notes
Notes
3rd Party Impressions

Season	Day/Night?
Occasion	Buy Again?

Projection ☆☆☆☆☆	Longevity ☆☆☆☆☆

Overall Rating ☆☆☆☆☆

Fragrance	
Brand	Location
Date	Cost

☐ Parfum ☐ Eau De Parum ☐ Eau De Toilette
☐ Eau De Cologne ☐ Eau Fraiche

Application?
Packaging
Initial Impression
Head/Top Notes
Heart/Middle Notes
Base Notes
Notes
3rd Party Impressions

Season	Day/Night?
Occasion	Buy Again?

Projection ☆☆☆☆☆	Longevity ☆☆☆☆☆

Overall Rating ☆☆☆☆☆

Fragrance	
Brand	Location
Date	Cost

☐ Parfum ☐ Eau De Parum ☐ Eau De Toilette
☐ Eau De Cologne ☐ Eau Fraiche

Application?
Packaging
Initial Impression
Head/Top Notes
Heart/Middle Notes
Base Notes
Notes
3rd Party Impressions

Season	Day/Night?
Occasion	Buy Again?
Projection ☆☆☆☆☆	Longevity ☆☆☆☆☆

Overall Rating ☆☆☆☆☆

Fragrance	
Brand	Location
Date	Cost

□ Parfum □ Eau De Parum □ Eau De Toilette
□ Eau De Cologne □ Eau Fraiche

Application?
Packaging
Initial Impression
Head/Top Notes
Heart/Middle Notes
Base Notes
Notes
3rd Party Impressions

Season	Day/Night?
Occasion	Buy Again?

Projection ☆☆☆☆☆	Longevity ☆☆☆☆☆

Overall Rating ☆☆☆☆☆

Fragrance	
Brand	Location
Date	Cost

☐ Parfum ☐ Eau De Parum ☐ Eau De Toilette
☐ Eau De Cologne ☐ Eau Fraiche

Application?	
Packaging	
Initial Impression	
Head/Top Notes	
Heart/Middle Notes	
Base Notes	
Notes	
3rd Party Impressions	

Season	Day/Night?
Occasion	Buy Again?

Projection ☆☆☆☆☆	Longevity ☆☆☆☆☆

Overall Rating ☆☆☆☆☆

Fragrance	
Brand	Location
Date	Cost

☐ Parfum ☐ Eau De Parum ☐ Eau De Toilette
☐ Eau De Cologne ☐ Eau Fraiche

Application?	
Packaging	
Initial Impression	
Head/Top Notes	
Heart/Middle Notes	
Base Notes	
Notes	
3rd Party Impressions	

Season	Day/Night?
Occasion	Buy Again?

Projection ☆☆☆☆☆	Longevity ☆☆☆☆☆

Overall Rating ☆☆☆☆☆

Fragrance	
Brand	Location
Date	Cost

☐ Parfum ☐ Eau De Parum ☐ Eau De Toilette
☐ Eau De Cologne ☐ Eau Fraiche

Application?
Packaging
Initial Impression
Head/Top Notes
Heart/Middle Notes
Base Notes
Notes
3rd Party Impressions

Season	Day/Night?
Occasion	Buy Again?

Projection ☆☆☆☆☆	Longevity ☆☆☆☆☆

Overall Rating ☆☆☆☆☆

Fragrance	
Brand	Location
Date	Cost

☐ Parfum ☐ Eau De Parum ☐ Eau De Toilette
☐ Eau De Cologne ☐ Eau Fraiche

Application?
Packaging
Initial Impression
Head/Top Notes
Heart/Middle Notes
Base Notes
Notes
3rd Party Impressions

Season	Day/Night?
Occasion	Buy Again?

Projection ☆☆☆☆☆	Longevity ☆☆☆☆☆

Overall Rating ☆☆☆☆☆

Fragrance	
Brand	Location
Date	Cost

☐ Parfum ☐ Eau De Parum ☐ Eau De Toilette
☐ Eau De Cologne ☐ Eau Fraiche

Application?
Packaging
Initial Impression
Head/Top Notes
Heart/Middle Notes
Base Notes
Notes
3rd Party Impressions

Season	Day/Night?
Occasion	Buy Again?

Projection ☆☆☆☆☆	Longevity ☆☆☆☆☆

Overall Rating ☆☆☆☆☆

Fragrance	
Brand	Location
Date	Cost

□ Parfum □ Eau De Parum □ Eau De Toilette
□ Eau De Cologne □ Eau Fraiche

Application?	
Packaging	
Initial Impression	
Head/Top Notes	
Heart/Middle Notes	
Base Notes	
Notes	
3rd Party Impressions	
Season	Day/Night?
Occasion	Buy Again?

Projection ☆☆☆☆☆	Longevity ☆☆☆☆☆

Overall Rating ☆☆☆☆☆

Fragrance	
Brand	Location
Date	Cost

☐ Parfum ☐ Eau De Parum ☐ Eau De Toilette
☐ Eau De Cologne ☐ Eau Fraiche

Application?	
Packaging	
Initial Impression	
Head/Top Notes	
Heart/Middle Notes	
Base Notes	
Notes	
3rd Party Impressions	

Season	Day/Night?
Occasion	Buy Again?

Projection ☆☆☆☆☆	Longevity ☆☆☆☆☆
Overall Rating ☆☆☆☆☆	

Fragrance	
Brand	Location
Date	Cost

☐ Parfum ☐ Eau De Parum ☐ Eau De Toilette
☐ Eau De Cologne ☐ Eau Fraiche

Application?
Packaging
Initial Impression
Head/Top Notes
Heart/Middle Notes
Base Notes
Notes
3rd Party Impressions

Season	Day/Night?
Occasion	Buy Again?

Projection ☆☆☆☆☆	Longevity ☆☆☆☆☆

Overall Rating ☆☆☆☆☆

www.ingramcontent.com/pod-product-compliance
Lightning Source LLC
Chambersburg PA
CBHW080600030426
42336CB00019B/3268